like a flower

like a flower

MY YEARS OF YOGA
WITH VANDA SCARAVELLI

Sandra Sabatini

with photographs by
Dr. David Darom

translated by
Ann Colcord

Like a Flower: My Years of Yoga with Vanda Scaravelli

First published in Great Britain by Pinter & Martin Ltd 2011

ISBN 978-1-905177-29-5

British Library Cataloguing-in-Publication Data
A catalogue record for this book is available from the British Library

Printed by Tien Wah Press Ltd, Singapore

Pinter & Martin Ltd
6 Effra Parade
London SW2 1PS

www.pinterandmartin.com

To all my travelling companions

contents

preface   11
meeting vanda   13
the first lesson   19
slowly   25
standing   31
the wave   35
sparks   39
that certain smile   45
like a flower   51
touch   57
between sky and ground   61
extraordinary lessons   67
yoga poses   75
a hymn to freedom   81
breath   85
treasure house   89
infinite time   95
epilogue: listening   101

photography   107
acknowledgements   108
about the author   109

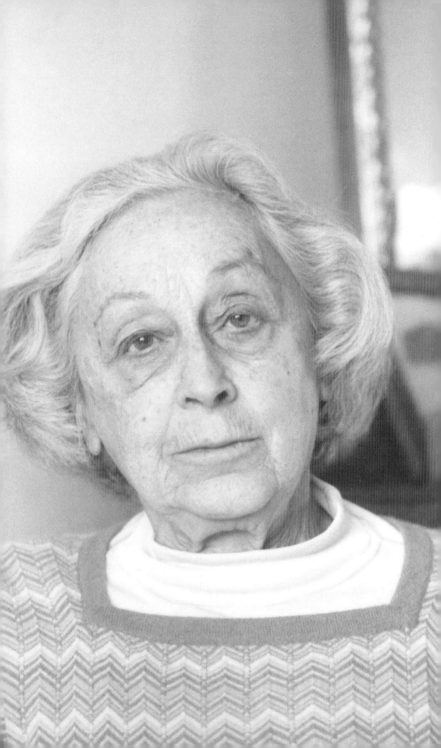

infinity

This lonely hill was ever dear to me
And this green hedge, that hides so large a part
Of the remote horizon from my view.
But as I sit and gaze, my mind conceives
Unending spaces, silences unearthly,
And deepest peace, wherein the heart almost
Draws nigh to fear. And as I hear the wind
Rustling among the branches, I compare
That everlasting silence with this sound:
Eternity is mine, and all past ages,
And this age living still, with all its noise.
So in immensity my thought is drowned,
And sweet it is to founder in this sea.

Giacomo Leopardi
L'Infinito from *I Canti* 1819-20
translated by Iris Origo

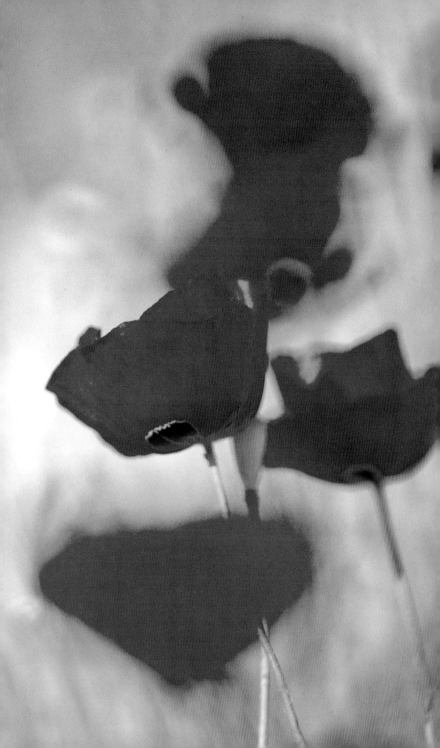

preface

My years of yoga with Vanda are wrapped in a gleam of light, like childhood memories and other special events, so that the memories remain untouched by the passing of time.

For many years I barely spoke about them with my students unless certain memories could add insights to the yoga practice. If that was the case I would extract a few of them from their protective bubble and later replace them very carefully.

I hope to enter that world of memories with great respect and love for those special years of studying with Vanda and at the end seal it up again, so it can go on glowing with that special luminosity for many years to come.

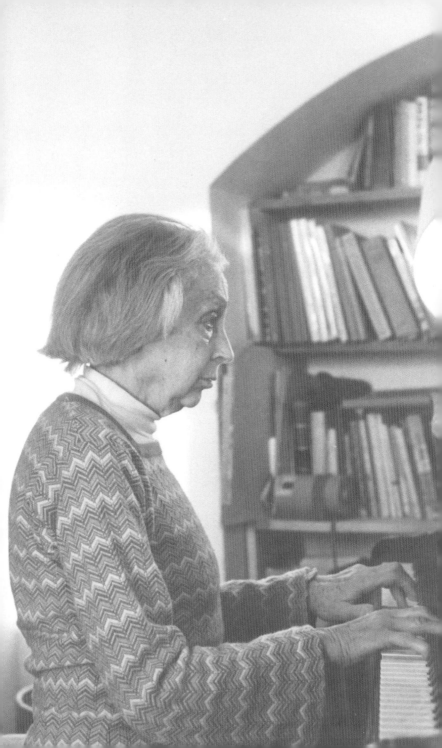

meeting vanda

I had heard of Vanda and her house from people who
had been invited to her Sunday lunches. On these
occasions, she used to gather friends and artists and
open her house to them. The house was situated a
few kilometres outside Florence on the hill of Fiesole.
It was surrounded by tall trees and overlooked the
beautiful valley of Mugnone.

When I was first invited to her house, it was to
celebrate my yoga teacher Dona Holleman's birthday,
and on that special occasion Dona brought some of
her students along.

At the time, Vanda was around 70 years old, a small woman with wonderful hands, very vivid eyes and white hair. From that visit, I learned that her remarks were always sharp, short and cleverly to the point. She did not enjoy long sentences or long conversations. It felt like she was very happy to offer her friends and guests the chance of meeting and she was very keen to provide time, food and beautiful surroundings. But she would never sit at the table for more than two minutes and often when you wished to talk to her she was nowhere to be found. Not in her house, not in the garden. To this day I wonder where she disappeared. And yet the few words you exchanged with her were like nectar, condensed. Intensity in its purest form.

At lunch, almost like magic, the doors to the dining room were opened. The table, almost three metres long, was laid with delicious food: lasagne, risotto, naked gnocchi, fresh eggs, salads and the most incredible variety of vegetables straight from the garden. Paola, the cook, had an extraordinary ability to present vegetables in so many different ways.

I think I saw Vanda several times like this – at a distance – and I was curious about the people who were coming and going with such nonchalance. Vanda once asked me about yoga and I told her I liked going to Dona's classes at a centre in via Ricasoli, and at the beginning I had signed up for one lesson a week, then two, then three, and now I was going to every course I could. Dona had then asked me to join a morning class with a group of advanced pupils who intended to become teachers one day that I was very happy to join.

As Dona's students we only visited Vanda occasionally, but Dona was having regular classes with Vanda, and I was struck by the fresh approach I glimpsed in her teaching.

When my daughter Chiara was born, and Michele three years later, I told Vanda about the birth at home, and how the yoga and breathing had not only been a great help, but a source of remarkable discoveries for me.

After their births, my body began to require a more subtle and attentive practice, and I felt that all the positions I had enjoyed before had lost their appeal, and I needed something different. My body refused to do complicated positions, but even in simple ones I found myself unnecessarily rigid. I felt more fragmented now than at the very beginning of my yoga practice, when my body was required to follow rules it refused to obey. I was waking up in the morning and finding that the moment I decided to move to my yoga mat my body was becoming painfully stiff. A high fever would follow this alarming state of stiffness, which indicated that something was very wrong.

I telephoned to say that I was at a crossroads. There had been frequent talk about going to India to study and acquire a diploma that would permit teaching in Europe.

Vanda suggested we meet in Florence and as soon as I sat on the sofa next to her I burst into tears. I didn't want to leave my three children and go to India to get a diploma. The only thing I knew for certain was that I needed a competent guide to help me out of all this confusion.

Tears kept flowing and Vanda kept handing me more tissues and then told me to go home and rest. I was puzzled and looked at her for a short time, and then she embraced me and literally shoved me out of the door. I was agitated and confused. I had three little children and a great love for yoga, but I didn't know how I could possibly choose between them.

Two days later Vanda telephoned to ask me to meet her at Fiesole. She said something very simple to me like "Vieni" which was neither a question nor an invitation. It was something completely unexpected which left me with the feeling of vast space as if I had been carried up to an improbable height. I believe I mumbled something like "When?" and "Yes, I'd be happy to". Probably no complete sentence was uttered that day.

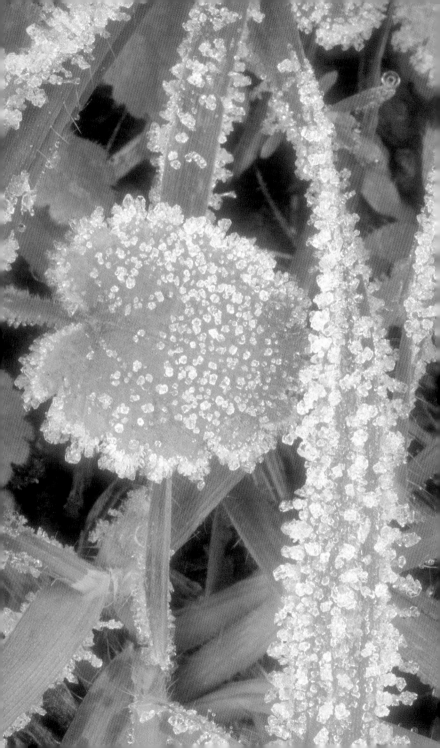

the first lesson

I was so overcome by powerful emotions that the trip to Fiesole, a few days later, brought out anxiety, nervousness, worry, and the continual question "What can I show her?" I was so utterly confused that I had forgotten I was going to Vanda to learn from her. I had anticipated showing her what yoga positions I had been learning and achieving. At that moment I still felt yoga was about showing prowess in the positions.

We sat on the sofa and she showed me a large calendar with photographs of Egyptian sculpture and drawings, enormous statues with straight spines, huge basalt feet with long toes, eyes elongated towards the temples and an authority that skimmed over the centuries to arrive directly at us. It seemed crucial, even from that first day, to understand the regal quality of those statues because they were the embodiment of the essence of yoga.

Vanda, sitting next to me, often said: "Guarda! Osserva! Pay attention to the feet, to the spine, the opening at the base of the skull and the space between the eyes." She saw in those works of art the proof of a physical awareness – a direct understanding of the connection with the sky and the earth.

Months later, on a visit to London, I spent some time at the British Museum placing myself in front of the statues to observe the movement. They were still walking, decisive and elegant, revealing vital energy in their gait. They let themselves be supported by the spine and let it lengthen towards the ground, towards the heels and then extended up towards the sky through the crown of the head.

I looked also at the back of the statues, and despite the basalt and marble, there was something alive, something that they felt compelled to represent – like a message to pass on – which Vanda had understood and was dedicated to transmitting to her students. That calendar image was frequently used in the coming years when Vanda wanted to emphasize the calm, authoritative, regal quality the Egyptians gave to the positions.

That day, at last, I asked something that was of crucial importance to me. I wanted to know if in her experience the choice of dedicating oneself to the study of yoga required a clean break, like a duty to leave everything behind. I told her I was very close to my three children and if yoga required that sort of sacrifice, I should have to renounce studying it. I had often heard people talk about yoga as a path that required total dedication and I wanted to learn her opinion before going on. Vanda stood up and went into the garden that surrounded her house, leaving me with the Egyptian Pharaohs who were looking at me, silent and serene. She returned half an hour later and told me that the study of yoga did not require such a drastic choice, but merely unlimited time and no ambition.

Years later she told me that at the time of our first meeting she had felt a total dedication was necessary but my question had made her think differently and she now felt that the desire to learn was all that was needed. Her response gave me a sense of well-being and serenity. We would have unlimited time before us, and nothing to keep us from plunging in. It sounded simple and possible.

For a long time, I had felt like a flower that had been hit by too many heavy drops of rain. Now it might recover some beauty in a very sunny warm climate.

We met then in the room where Vanda taught, which had a grand piano, a bed and a large bookshelf up to the ceiling. The room looked out over the valley of Fiesole, a valley covered with olive trees, and always basking in the sun. I felt nervous and eager to please her; I wanted to show her that I would be an excellent student. She pointed out a yoga mat on the ground and a blanket and told me to lie down and bend my knees. She put her huge feet on mine, several times; she used a firm and precise hold to lengthen the base of my skull and my neck. She placed her long pianist's fingers on my forehead and on my eyes, and asked me to breathe, slowly, without hurry and without effort. I think I produced a series of suffocated sounds because

Vanda repeated the words several times: "slowly, gently, without rushing and without effort".

These concepts were so unknown that it took me a long time to be able to go along with them. She had placed her hand on my abdomen and pushed it down lightly with each exhalation. That simple touch made me aware of how to shift attention and this made me even more nervous. Vanda repeated the same message with a dry and decisive voice: "breathe slowly, without rushing and without effort." But I anticipated the movement of her hand and forgot to inhale, so I exhaled in little huffs and puffs. I don't remember how many weeks Vanda made me spend on that yoga mat – probably until she saw some glimpse of letting go, until she felt a breath that could be given that name.

I remember that when I left that first session, I was aware of having found a guide of remarkable clarity, pure as a diamond, but my whole being was rebelling at this demanding and determined guidance. I very much liked the place where she had brought me, but I didn't have any sense of being able to get there on my own and sometimes even doubted that it truly existed, it was so fleeting and ephemeral.

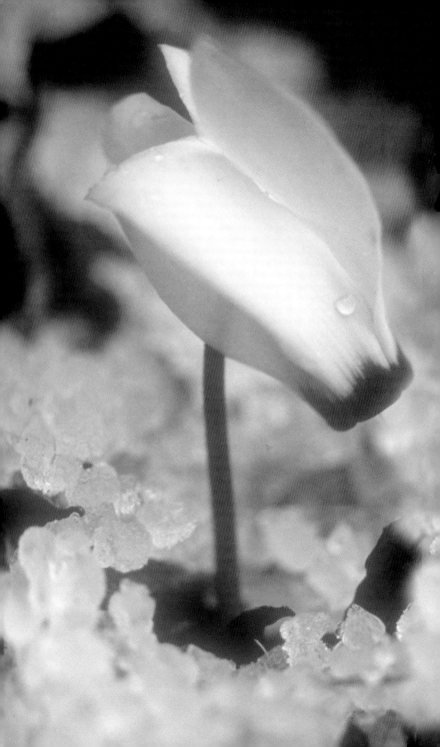

slowly

Slowly and gradually something infinitely tiny began to change. There was the breath – actually it was the exhalation and also the inhalation. They followed each other without pauses or ceasing, and they existed together. Sometimes I couldn't even distinguish one from the other. There was also the ground below me which sent reassuring messages. It could support me and I could entrust myself to its solidity. One day, I finally relaxed enough to fully sink into the ground. It felt as if I were the first woman to land on the moon, and while my body was sinking on the yoga mat, a white and very fine, light dust arose around me. This was a small miracle. It was very hard to let myself go, listen to her words, follow her suggestions. I felt weak and was often tired of listening. I wanted to escape from that voice that was pointing out things that were precise but not understood.

That first day and for many other meetings, I was glad that Vanda was reassuring me of the simplicity of the path we were following, and using poetic images. But she must have been aware of how hard and tiresome it was for me to listen to my continuous, senseless inner tumult. It was so noisy and congested.

Every week I telephoned to ask her if "my day" was free. Sometimes the phrase seemed to twist itself around and Vanda would then ask me to call her the following day. Sometimes she could hear the tiredness in my voice, and suggested I stay at home and rest. Occasionally she told me the time was not right: too cold, too hot, too rainy. Sometimes I tried to prepare the questions to ask her, in order to get a positive response: "Yes, do come". She tended to sense my actual state of mind and would postpone any decision to the following day.

I tried not to lose heart, because I had read about masters who put their students to the test, and perhaps Vanda was testing my patience. In every remark of hers I found a seed of wisdom and of truth that encouraged me to persist in my practice even if I was not able to meet her.

Whenever she said yes, I flew up to Fiesole in a state of exhilaration. Once in the course of a telephone call she said "Come with your heart, that is all that matters." I had wanted to tell her my heart was so full of love for this meeting that she had created a feverish state in me.

Very often on my way to Vanda's house by car, I was startled at the sight of a bizarre being in the distance, walking by the side of the road. Winter or summer, the disguise was always the same: wrapped up in a blue woollen jacket, enormous dark sun glasses which covered the whole face, black leggings and a pair of white flipflops. This mysterious creature was walking slowly, spending a long time in each and every step, with hands – palms together – behind her. Every time it took me a few minutes to recognize my teacher.

One day when I arrived at her house, I opened the door of her room and couldn't see the yoga mat and the blanket. After months of positions on the floor we had moved on to the standing or mountain pose: tadasana. The toes extend out from the foot, the heels sink into the ground and the outsides of the feet are well anchored to the ground. In this deceptively simple position, I often felt exhausted, like a flower that has reclined its corolla, slightly lopsided and unable to find its verticality.

Vanda placed her feet on mine, then she sat down on the floor, aligned the outside of my feet, pressed my heels into the ground, held my calves with her hands and shook me and shoved me from right to left. She sometimes pushed me off my centre of gravity, to give me a different sense of balance, lower, more towards the back of the body. With her clear and precise voice she repeated: "Relax, let go, let the weight drop into the ground, feel the roots, breathe, there is no hurry".

Her touch was forceful and compelling. I had the feeling of being deconstructed by her hands in order to be recomposed in a new form, more elastic and more spacious. Her hands had an extraordinary incisiveness: they penetrated and found space in those hidden places between the toes, behind the shoulder blades, at the back of the knees, between the vertebrae of the neck, where the spine joins the base of the skull, behind the ears, in the centre of the feet, in the palm of the hands. They worked incessantly and diligently and seemed to have a life of their own and multiply into thousands. They could enter and wake up and create space where it had not existed before.

Often with closed eyes, to listen better to what she was saying, I had the feeling that her hands had multiplied and also her feet, her touch had propagated itself all over the surface of my body.

From the state of total disorientation when I had first met Vanda, I felt that I was beginning to feel the good effects of her continual references to the ground, to the spine and to the breath. Contact with the ground I found comforting, and my breathing was improving. I was able to be less brusque and aggressive in my practice. I was still hearing peremptory orders from the past that related to this or that position, but now I was opening my eyes and the hands of Vanda guided me towards a dimension of receptivity, listening and calm.

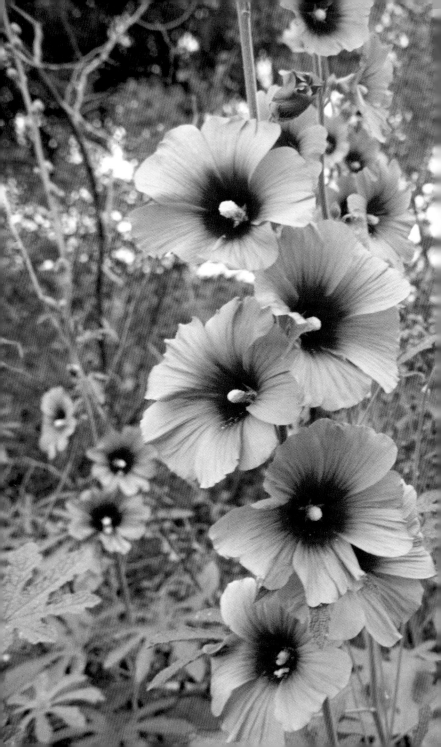

standing

In this position, the feet show up all the poor habits of posture. In fact it is not considered so much a position but a transition point or passageway. If you are lacking a wall for support you tend to lean on one side and then the other, curving the waist, arching the spine, making it become something unsustainable.

Vanda often stressed the importance and value of the mountain pose, saying that when it was experienced fully you understood all that there was to learn about yoga positions. Mountain pose is full of tiny and subtle shifts that rise up from the feet towards the head. It can be like a miniature earthquake that upsets any restrictive twist the body may have settled into. It is these postural weaknesses, twists and strange curves in the spine, and ways of standing and moving that have all imprinted themselves on the body, making the position difficult and tiring to maintain.

Mountain pose as Vanda taught it is truly revolutionary. The feet are parallel and kept apart to free the pelvis of excessive weight. The toes are extended and long, and the weight is shifted gradually back towards the heels. Vanda spoke often of eyes behind the knees, and also eyes under the feet or in the centre of the hands, eyes that brought vitality and attention to places that were often neglected.

For the first few months I found practising mountain pose very tiring, but then I moved into a state of greater calm and a deeper listening. Helped by Vanda's hands, I managed to bring my attention to the bottom of the feet and to breathe towards the soles and slowly develop a sense of roots even in a rudimentary state.

I was also learning the importance of being present and participating in all the small adjustments that take place in the course of the practice, not that I always succeeded. But I was beginning to get glimpses of the incredible intelligence that this active presence released. Maybe the origin of so much of my tightness and contraction, strains and pains was the lack of this continual attention. In feeling the breath reach down to the feet, the weight shifts towards the heels, and the body, instead of losing balance, extends the toes and finds a new alignment in a sinuous movement that frees the body from a great deal of rigidity.

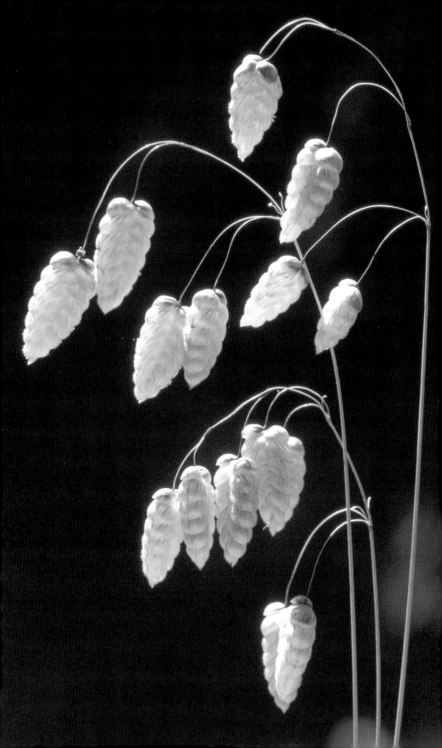

the wave

After the first months when Vanda had guided me towards a state of greater relaxation and capacity to listen she began to speak of the wave. At the beginning I had thought "What a beautiful image". All images from nature are powerful and speak directly to the body in its own language, but I knew that Vanda would also stay by my side, day by day, for months and if necessary for years until my own body had sensed the wave, until my body had become that wave.

The feet relax in contact with the ground, the breath arrives all the way to the feet, the centre of gravity shifts back when the heels sink into the ground. The shoulders then become light and the head as well, so that when the breath enters the body there is much more space to move into and more lightness in which to expand.

You feel taller, with a new space around your waist, extending from the waist down because it is drawn by the force of gravity. But you are also drawn upwards from the waist by the space above.

When I felt the wave move through me for just a fraction of a second, I felt rewarded for all the effort I had made when I had been asked to abandon myself to the breath and to the force of gravity. It had been a painstaking task to bring the tiny fragments of a mosaic together into a composition. The breath, the spine, the feet, the ground, the sky and the scattered fragments needed to be gathered together but also needed a delicate and vibrant understanding like a ray of sunshine to continually illuminate the practice. When this happens, you find yourself in a precise place, luminous and sparkling, full of joy.

Sometimes Vanda and I sat together on a sunny stone step and tried to describe this place – 'joy', perhaps or 'happiness' or 'allegrezza'. The English word 'bliss' seemed to get close, but euphoria or a diffuse state of lovingness were also part of the feeling. In the end we usually agreed that this unique place could not be described in words and this safeguarded its beauty and uniqueness. It was a quality of attention delicate and light as a butterfly that marked every breath and every slight interior change without pressure, and without pausing more than a second. And that light touch was more than enough to lead you into new and pristine spaces.

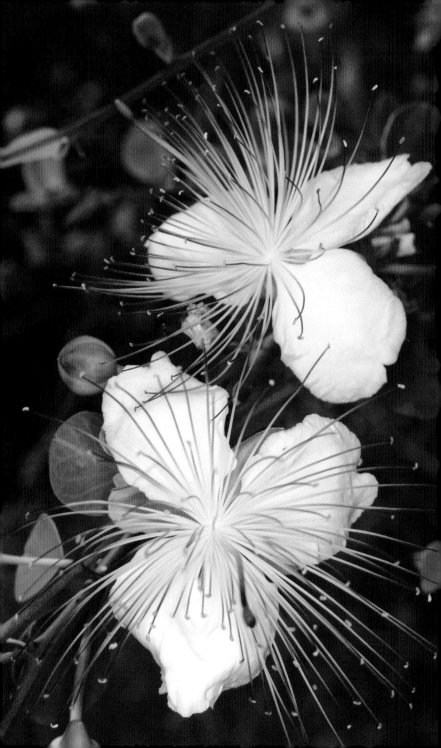

sparks

Vanda used to say that yoga took hold of you by the hairs of your head, imperiously, and you had to go along because there seemed no choice. In effect, the echo left by every session stayed for days and days, often showing new significance and fresh possibilities.

At night the body continued to release, and sometimes in unexpected jerks, and at times a burning feeling in the soles of my feet would wake me up. During the day it was sometimes necessary to lie down and stretch out, or go out for a walk to allow another in a series of infinite interior adjustments to find their place.

Her voice and her steady touch encouraged a feeling of becoming more alive. My entire being seemed to vibrate until it reached a new balance where it could then fall into a deep and restorative sleep, and sometimes the following day I would find myself walking in a way that felt completely new. There seemed no end to the capacity to let the roots grow more deeply into the ground, nor to sensing the lengthening wave that linked the ground and the sky and the expansion that followed.

It seemed astonishing to discover that the positions and certain practices with the breath brought me to different places every time. Vanda's insights brought a release not only from muscular tensions but also from habitual patterns of thought. For example I had previously learned that alignment demanded a precise symmetry, but Vanda never suggested that. She recommended finding a solid base through the feet that was neither rigid nor fixed so that when the force of gravity became more active, the body could free itself in an undulating movement which created its own alignment, and all from within. It was like a green bamboo stalk and the nodes were places where movement could pass. It was a chance to transform oneself into a blade of grass swaying in the breeze without losing the roots, or a flower of amazing shades of red bathing in the warmth of the sun.

Another concept I was holding onto which melted like snow in the sun's rays concerned maintaining the positions: staying in a position for a certain amount of time. What happened to me before was that instead of listening to the breath and favouring the state of deep peace, I had been shifting my attention onto staying in the position, bringing in an element of force which had disrupted the harmony and simplicity.

Vanda seemed to push you more deeply inside the position with her hands and her voice, so the body felt absolutely centred, aided by the force of gravity and the natural need to expand. It was like finding a friendly place where there was only a precise instant of disarming clarity. An extraordinary sense of well-being and lightness arose. You felt different, as if you had shed heavy, old and dusty clothes and were in a state where the physical yielded to a diffused luminosity. Her guidance demanded an utter compliance without ever feeling a need to define the purpose of the practice.

Once I asked her if this was a spiritual practice and the silence that followed was so full of question marks that I didn't want to ask again. Those kinds of questions either fell into the void or she would say something dry and dismissive like "It doesn't matter". This process of cutting dead the development of some inference or theory left me disoriented. I needed something I could hold on to which would sustain me in following the practice, but everything I tried to hold on to seemed to be pulled away from me before I could grasp it. Was it just a matter of loving the practice in every moment, and nothing more?

From the moment I entered her room, perhaps from the time I knocked at the door, I felt that I could leave everything else behind and respond fully to her suggestions. As I began to acquire "the art of shedding everything" when I arrived at Vanda's, I became impatient to begin the session. Every moment lost was a vast loss and so it was for Vanda. It is true that there was infinite time before us but there was also urgency in getting back to that state of listening, that I perceived as a compelling need to meet her and begin the session. I felt I was always starting from the beginning.

Vanda never claimed to be one who knew, or understood secrets that would one day be revealed. There was the sense that everything was already there waiting for the student who merely had to get in contact with the ground and the space through the spine. The breath would bring it all together.

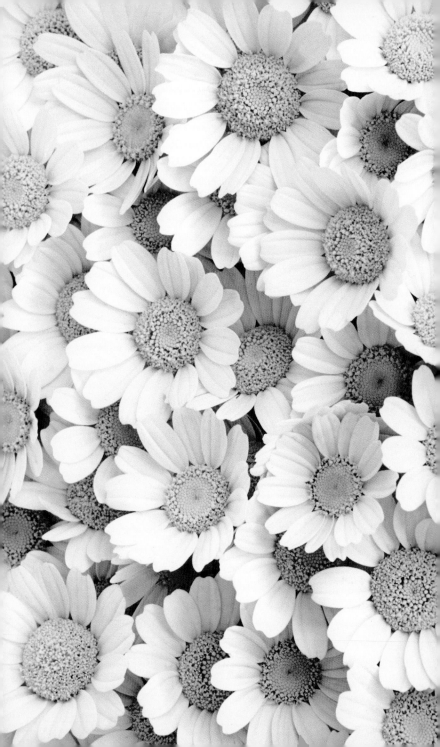

that certain smile

In some photographs in her book *Awakening the Spine* there is a smile that ripples the corners of her mouth and makes her eyes gleam with naughtiness. It appears whenever she wants to persuade you that what she is saying is easy to do, very easy. It may be associated with a particularly difficult position that Vanda would assure you was very simple and then only minutes later advise you never to try.

At other times, the smile appears with a breathing practice and she would say "Pay attention to the exhalation, and all the rest will take care of itself." The smile reassures you that there is some truth in her words, but that she hopes you would understand that there are infinite steps for you to take in order to get there.

On other occasions she would claim "There are no teachers nor students. We are all teachers and students at the same time." Then again a certain crinkle in her face opens into a smile that warns you with infinite benevolence that the road is long but there are already tracks that could be followed with simplicity and faithfulness.

When she said to me once that there were not two roads but always and only a single one, her eyes brightened at my look of perplexity. "What, aren't there two roads and one has to choose a single one?" No, said her smile, and it was a smile warmly human and slightly teasing. She created a suspension of time in the air, a pause which gave you the chance to reflect on her words. That pause produced a change, like an internal somersault, suddenly revealing that single road showing itself right in front of you.

But the most splendid smile I received was when I returned from a seminar on vedic chanting. From the very first day of the seminar I had felt out of place. I was experiencing a general feeling of distress which developed into a high fever that persisted throughout the night. I dreamed that a young woman asked me what yoga truly might be and where it could be found. In the dream I showed her the ocean in all its vastness and the seabed near the shore, places with rocks and a sandy bottom and pavings of thick seaweed and clear tranquil water. For me, I told her, yoga is represented by the ocean and the wave that arises out of it, an iridescent wave that ascends many metres out of the sea and then crashes down into the water below, creating thousands of ripples.

Next time I met her, I told Vanda that during the workshop, I came across a very definite discovery: I felt how her teachings had filled up every little corner of my being, to such an extent that there was no physical space for anything else. Not in my heart, not anywhere else. Then her face opened into the most luminous of her smiles.

In the course of her years of practice Vanda had come into contact with something precious. She had come upon yoga by chance, as she used to say, and it had taken her down an unexpected road, with no final destination. Now the time had come to transmit it with the clarity of one who had practised almost as a pastime, without ever wishing to teach, and then quite by chance to friends and acquaintances.

That certain smile speaks of a precise vision she had attained and felt ready to share with others. She wished to introduce a sense of listening into yoga practice and a keen attention that accompanied the student every minute and avoided any harsh or abrupt movements. Too often she saw people who had damaged themselves in their practice and it was hard to reconcile a joyful and beautiful experiment like yoga with aches and pains and damaged joints. Attention to the breath offered a safeguard and brought gentleness. Circular movements let the body release and move. The smile says there is a great deal to discover in the course of life and that is what makes this road such a fascinating one.

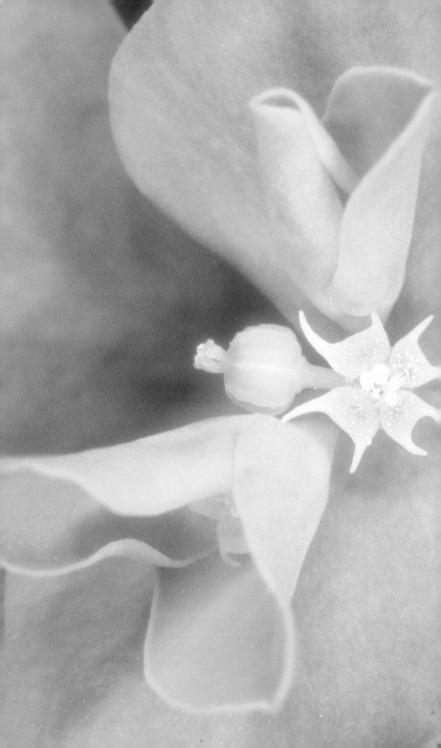

like a flower

Vanda often said that a revolution was needed to restore yoga to its essence. Her radical approach required continual awareness of all that is going on inside from the moment we begin to discern that gravity is everywhere. Although it has no colour or flavour or sound, gravity is the most pervasive force in the human habitat. It is true that we unwittingly resist it all our lives. Vanda taught that when we become aware of it, gravity becomes an ally, a resource we can call upon, and the gift to discover and learn how to use it should not be confused with any other gift. We experience it internally, it cannot be photographed or copied, but it is a remarkable experience every time we sense it and feel it.

From this contact with the ground Vanda drew inspiration to guide us and awaken in each of us the wish to play with the sense of gravity every time we came to an exhalation. Vanda often used the image of a flower and showed them to me growing brightly coloured and innocent in the fields around her house. To become like a flower that grows out of the ground, gets longer, blossoms and slowly withers. Silent as a flower, beautiful, modest as a flower, with that indescribable movement of opening from the centre, revealing all the beauty enclosed within.

This opening of petals is the movement that we meet in the palm of the hand, on the sole of the feet, at the top of the head and in other centres of our body when the breath and the awareness touch. It is the movement that accompanies us every time we allow ourselves to open, trusting in the new.

Every time Vanda reminded me of the existence of this movement I felt a thick blanket of sounds and whispers slide away from my head and shoulders leaving me lighter. It was a re-entry into the stream of life, innocent like a flower and out of time. "You see," she would say, "Flowers are never hurried but they grow in thousands of different shapes and colours. We should be like them."

Vanda loved nature and references to its beauty were essential for me, I heard the force of her words because they spoke of something familiar: rivers, flowers, the sea, the wave, the sky, that connection with the surroundings gave the practice truth and vitality. A poetic language which evoked familiar objects. There was no superstructure nor inventions nor secrets in her teaching. Everything could be attained and explored by the light of day. For years, before I met her, I stiffened whenever yoga was presented as a series of secret steps which could not be divulged until the time was right. Vanda's images showed a disarming simplicity that brought me back to being a beginner again, curious and keen to learn over and over again.

The flower's roots lengthen within the earth and become strong and tenacious to allow what is above to expand into space, seeking light. Using a few concise phrases, under Vanda's guidance, the body felt it was flowering, happy to be in contact with mother earth and confident of being able to grow vertically. Then something opened within the verticality that could be called petals which meekly unfold creating the play of light and shade. The wind, or perhaps it was the breath, ruffled the petals and gently shook the leaves.

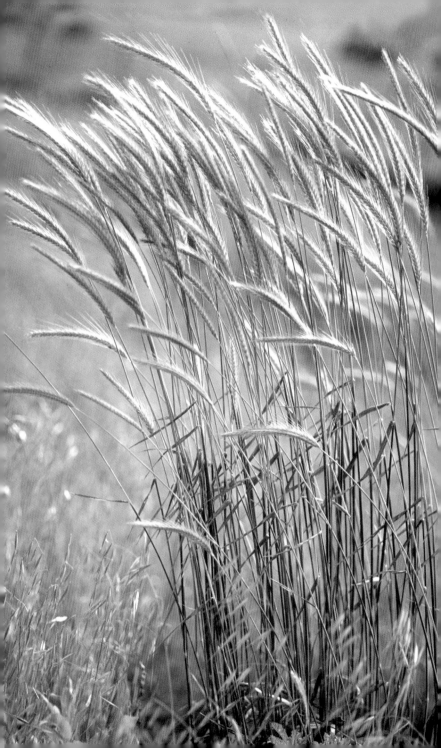

touch

For years I have been searching for words that could describe Vanda's hands and the way she used them when she touched her students during the yoga sessions. Her touch was, for me, a revelation.

After years of yoga where the instructor's forceful corrections created uneasiness and fear, the way Vanda used her hands to guide or help understand a pose, gave my body a natural impulse towards an innate and happy alignment. I never felt that there was a technique to be learned from her. She had an empathy with the student and an amazing ability to reach places of 'holding' – zeroing in on them with her eyes as well as her hands. Most of the time it felt like her hands were attracted by the well-hidden pockets of tension. There was no thinking involved, just a primal understanding of the body and an intuitive, loving way to relate deeply to the student.

With the students who had been through operations or were in pain, her touch was very careful. In these cases, the practice itself was especially relaxing and slow. I felt that she would stay and witness the natural healing process even if it took years.

"There is no hurry, do not rush" she would repeat like a modern mantra. With long-term students, her hands were demanding as if she wanted the outer, holding shield to break down, and in an even later stage, to dispel new tensions before they could cling and get encrusted. "Let go and surrender."

She knew how to use her hands without upsetting the students. By the way she did it, you felt that it was not an imposition but an act of love. Love and humility. The deep humility in Vanda's approach is all enclosed in three words: earth, feet, breath. She would direct attention to these elements, urging her students to develop a dialogue with them.

This humility is like a diamond, hard and clear. It is an essential state to be in every time you practise and every time you guide someone else.

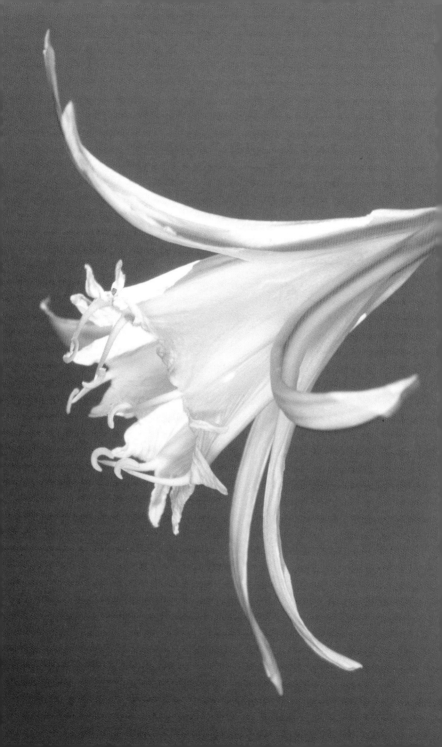

between sky and ground

The backbend from standing is a synthesis of the yoga Vanda was sharing with her students. Starting with tadasana, the mountain pose, experimenting with the different adjustments this position requires, and experiencing the shifts and changes needs continual alertness. Tadasana was for Vanda the pose that most encouraged what was going on in one's body when properly grounded.

The ground and gravity that one feels through the ground, and the space around us, are actual presences which not only inspire movement but are active and can be felt physically. It is our task to back them up with our breath.

The standing pose, with its smaller and more precarious base of support, invites an unexpected range of movements and changes. From moment to moment, from breath to breath, the body needs to adjust as it goes on dropping any kind of holding.

The position passes through different beginning stages of inevitable resistance and stiffness until it finally releases in a rhythmical contact with the ground that lets you bounce back gracefully upwards until the spine itself wants to bend backwards. When the legs have become utterly solid, gradually go down the wall or even in the centre of the room – all the way to the ground – before coming up again, like a wave that moves through the air with its beauty.

Often I would arrive at Fiesole to find Vanda, standing about a metre away from the wall using tiny rotating movements in her wrists to free her shoulders. She would visibly grow and lengthen. Her feet would respond to each exhalation and become very large, the heels sinking into the ground, her knees opening, and she was ready to receive the wave that led her upwards and then let her bend backwards.

This position made her very happy and she enjoyed explaining how easy it was while she did it. The exhalation reinforced her base, lengthened her roots below the ground and she gathered the contrary movement which arose from the ground upwards and confirmed the desire of the spine for lightness which led it to bend backwards spontaneously. Nothing more. And she smiled at this obvious simplicity.

Just watching her for a short time was enough to become convinced that nothing could be more simple or more easy than this practice. There was no sign of effort, neither in lengthening down to the ground nor in coming up into the starting position. Sometimes when she was going down and slowly coming up again she roused an irresistible wish to become barefoot and do what she was doing.

You would discover that the so-called 'simplicity' was the fruit of a long process of gradual releasing of tensions, where the breath could become gradually longer, the muscles could release and you could find a sublime absorption in the harmonious interplay between the ground and the sky. A single dimension within which the breath and the movement could harmonize under an attentive and benevolent watch.

The rhythm could be caught. It was released every time the exhalation reached the ground and arrived at the arch of the foot which, once it was open, was able to transmit the push that soared from on high down towards the ground, and then arose through the calf, opened the knee, reached the hip where it could then soar up the whole spine, mounting vertebra to vertebra until it broadened the base of the skull into a smile, then moved to the top at the crown of the head.

This continual alternating of exhalation towards the ground and inhalation which frees and lightens the upper part of the body creates an interior wave that encourages every segment of the body to move sinuously.

In the practice the backbend from standing reawakens the entire being because it is brought into a dimension of evolutionary growth and while in the other positions this movement seems barely sketched out, here it becomes ample and develops into an entire song.

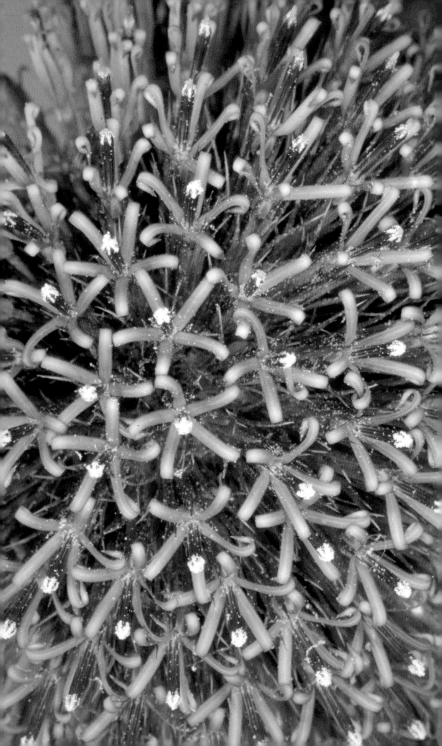

extraordinary lessons

Vanda always emphasized the need to stay alert without getting distracted or losing time. Driving a car on a rainy day was an ideal time for her to count the movements of the windscreen wiper, from left to right and from right to left, breathing in the rhythm of the wipers – this made the journey more restful.

The half-hour bus journey between Fiesole and Florence was also a good time to practise. When all the seats were full, a pole at the end of the bus was, for Vanda, an excellent prop for stretching and elongating the spine. In the course of this brief journey I found myself pushed by her against the pole, with her fist that methodically pressed my navel backward, with every exhalation. I had to ignore any surprised looks from the passengers and attend to the rhythmical encouragement of her voice: inhale, exhale, touch with your waist. Inhale, exhale, touch with your waist for the whole journey, as there was no time to lose.

Vanda's shopping expeditions in the centre of Florence were also good occasions to help people. She would invite any saleswomen who were haughtily walking on high heels to take off their shoes and find their centre of gravity again. She showed them how to release the toes, especially the fourth and fifth toes and assured them their backache would vanish. "First of all learn to stand, and breathe, keep breathing and you'll see how soon you'll feel better." And then she would go out with her purchase under her arm, as if blown by the wind.

If a group of students came to see her, she would start to teach right away, taking them by the hand and showing them how to walk, slowly, step after step, touching the ground with the heel, letting the foot spread, the toes stretching, and noticing how the back foot, secured by the roots, obliges the body to lengthen upwards. There was no time to waste because the revolution could not be put off; it needed to happen now, when the body, by trying out another dimension, felt a sudden sense of well-being.

In her generosity, she felt an urge to help whenever she saw someone in distress. Anyone who was suffering a stiff neck was immediately asked to lie on the ground so Vanda could use her skilled and decisive touch to lengthen the spine, stretch and dissolve that painful place. With knee problems Vanda's fingers would move to those two mysterious hollows in the back of the knee, and stay there for some time, burrowing more deeply inwards. Then her hands would move down to the heels to lengthen and release the contraction. The pain vanished and the knee was free.

A headache was soothed by stroking the temples in horizontal lines that released the skin on the forehead and put light pressure on the bony rim of the eye sockets. Little rotations of the head to the right and the left, her fingers probing the bones at the base of the skull as deeply as possible. She touched the chin and jaw to be sure it was released, and pushed the sternum down and continued to lengthen the neck.

If someone had a stiff back with pains in the shoulder, Vanda explained the need to pay attention to the heels when walking. "Spread the foot, position the heel so that the front of the ankle can open. Slowly, with small steps, you need to feel the foot sink in to the ground when you are walking, do you really feel it?" She made the person repeat the movement until she saw the right movement and, taking hold of the student's wrist, lengthen it down towards the ground, with the force of every exhalation.

If someone asked her about the breath she asked them to stretch out on the ground, and would lengthen them with emphatic movements. She then sat next to them and at every exhalation placed her big hand over the navel and pushed, asking them to produce the sound HA! "You see, the navel has to touch the ground when you exhale. Then it relaxes completely and receives the air. That's all it needs to do, receive the air."

I remember a student who wanted to learn to do a backbend from the ground. Vanda kept her breathing on the ground for almost an hour with her knees bent. At every exhalation her hand pushed the abdomen down to the ground and towards the tailbone with a precise and knowing movement. "That's good. Now you can come up with the next exhalation, but only at the end of the exhalation." The student rose up effortlessly into the most soaring backbend of her life.

If external distractions occurred during our yoga classes, she would turn it into a lesson about concentration. I remember a breathing lesson, interrupted when the plumber came to repair a bathroom pipe next to Vanda's teaching room. At one point he needed to use a very powerful drill, and Vanda in the deafening sound of drilling adjacent to us continued to whisper in my ear: "Inhale, exhale, inhale, exhale". Or another time when I arrived at her house for our weekly meeting to find the place in turmoil, with people coming and going in and out of her room. The woods nearby had caught fire, the firemen were about to arrive, and Vanda was sitting cross-legged in the centre of the room breathing imperturbably. After about fifteen minutes she stood up with her great smile and said to me: "Sandra, it is very important to continue breathing."

I remember once we were watching the flight of a falcon, with its claws pointing towards the ground when it was descending, its wings wide open. And I still have a faded and crumpled photograph of the bronchial tree, to help me identify with the expansion of the lungs during the breathing. One day there also appeared a strange yellow sponge which she put in my hand to re-create and help me understand the contraction and expansion of the lungs during breathing practice.

At other times I arrived with one of my children and she pulled out a big box which contained wooden building blocks, coloured cubes and books. Vanda arranged it all on a carpet close to the child so she could play and then began to focus on yoga practice. "If we can't pay attention to our breathing with a playing child next to us, then what is yoga all about?" After a meeting with her, before going home, she offered me many treats for the whole family: ravioli, polenta, pizza, fresh eggs, various vegetables. She wanted my day with her to be completely restful.

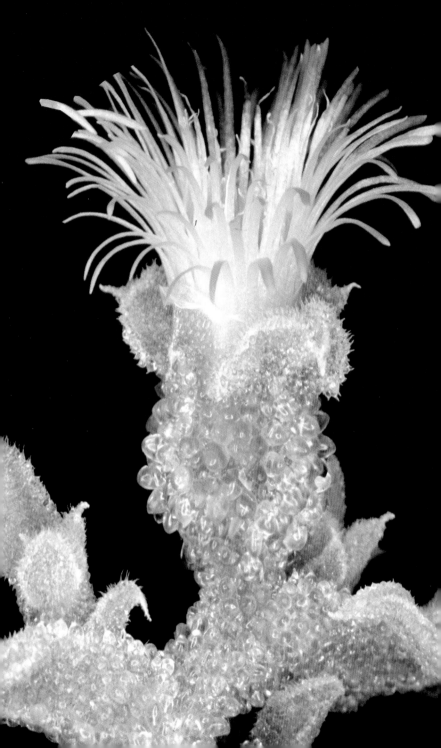

yoga poses

Vanda was very grateful to B.K.S. Iyengar for having introduced her to so many beautiful poses. She had a normal body and worked on undoing its resistance in order to achieve flexibility. It amused her to practise positions that were considered difficult. She was so solidly rooted to the ground and linked to the force of gravity that she could move in and out of any position without effort. She spoke of the poses as if they were amusing variously coloured toys that delighted her.

Her practice had great variety: she did the full range of the standing poses, the seated poses with the forward movement, all the variations of the backbends and the inverted poses. She used the same strategy for all of them: inhale, exhale, feel the part of the body in contact with the ground becoming totally anchored to the earth, and from there it lengthens, grows and extends in the opposite direction. Let the body lean backwards or forwards or sideways without hurry or effort.

In the last years she tended to prefer a long preparation of the mountain pose and then, close to a wall, a slow descent to the ground in a marvellous backbend. She would then come up again with utter grace. With the addition of some forward bends, it seemed to have become her favourite pose

She used a handsome eighteenth-century chest of drawers with the top drawer pulled out about a metre for help with a balancing pose on one leg with the back leg raised to represent Shiva while dancing. To watch her practice was always a source of inspiration, with her slight smile, bright eyes and continual challenge to time. I felt an irresistible urge to adopt the special joy and lightness she showed while practising, the fruit of many years of listening. The message her practice transmitted was unequivocal: "It is amusing, but this is not the place to stop, let's keep looking, and there is no end to discovery."

She used to say: "Once the fundamental principles of a strong base, the breath, the space and the vitality of the spine have been found, you can explore any position you please."

The poses were all pleasant because each of them invited you to play. There was something extremely childlike about the way Vanda approached them, and something vital that she released when she was practising. One day I asked: "What is this effervescence?" She smiled at me and said, "Energy". It was the only time in eighteen years I heard her use that word. She refused to use any definitions and any artificiality, as if they were poison. The Sanskrit names for the poses had, in the course of the years, either vanished or become so transformed they were unrecognisable. She reduced everything to the essential. To be freed from the names of the poses gave me a sense of freedom because it allowed me to encounter them as if for the first time, without even a name I could hold on to. To watch her practise was to witness a true hymn to freedom.

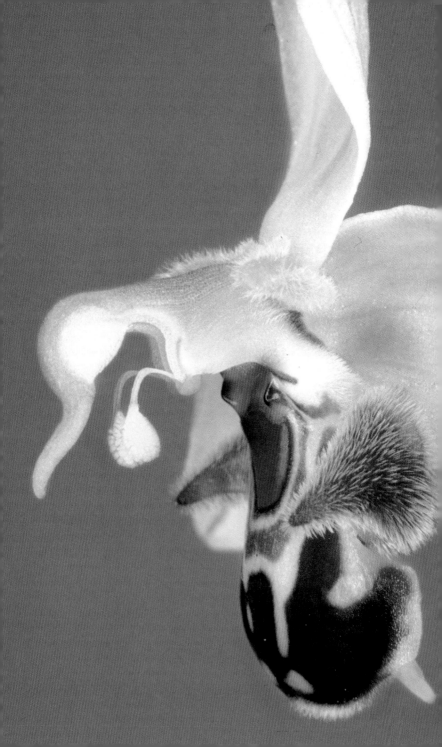

a hymn to freedom

What I sensed in the air that first day at Vanda's house was what I would now understand as the sense of freedom. It was part of the atmosphere at her house, in her friends and acquaintances, and it certainly showed in her. It was part of her steady openness with no useless encumbrances, her capacity to glide towards a serene attitude of paying attention with no distractions.

In her clarity and the essence of her being, and her long friendship with Krishnamurti, there was the same sense of freedom. The pathways marked by Krishnamurti and Vanda had much in common. A very subtle line along which to move – keeping your balance but with no illusions or certainties to hang on to.

It began with a lesson in clarity with no sense of authority or instruction. Both Krishnamurti and Vanda shunned the trap of authority. They both emphasized the importance of moving slowly so as to observe the way thoughts were moving. Reading Krishnamurti's books and watching some videos of his conferences I realized that they recreated for me a state of attentive listening quite beyond a normal intellectual curiosity.

I found the same sensation with Vanda. Her alert presence encouraged and elicited a full response or a presence equally alive and complete: an imperious request to shake off sleepiness and reawaken to the moment.

Vanda was capable of making concrete instructions to bring about what Krishnamurti proposed in his talks. It was as if Krishnamurti had prepared the road and Vanda had paved it with her intuitions – gravity, the spine, the breath. Both had found the way towards an inner silence, because only inner silence lets one regain innocence and freshness to live life in its entirety. Without ambitions, without great effort.

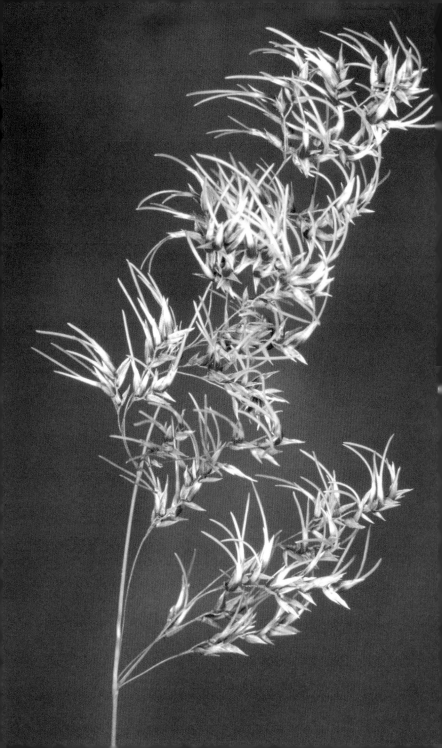

breath

One day when Vanda invited T.K. Desikachar and his
wife together with some of her pupils, Desikachar
chanted some Vedic hymns, which were beautiful.
At one point Vanda stood up and went to observe
him closely. Returning to her pupils a few minutes
later, very happy, she said that Desikachar's spine was
vibrating from top to tail during the chanting.

With her hands which touched various places while I
was breathing she had taught me more than countless
books. "Notice", she used to say, "It seems that there
is no more air to get rid of, but it is possible to get rid

of even more without effort. It is in that emptiness that we've created that the inhalation can come." Lying on the ground, or seated, or standing her fist that she placed just above the navel giving a downward movement reminded me to exhale deeply.

For years we remained with that essential practice, and then we passed on to breathing with a sound. Her favourite was Kapalabhati: the breath of the shining skull. It brought clarity and the whole day seemed to unfold before you without obstacles or any effort. Another favourite of hers was the vibrating breath. Seated facing me, she would press my knees to the ground, encouraging the legs to drop and she shook me to let my spine vibrate. Sometimes she extended her legs over mine to add extra weight. If all this attention didn't bring the result she hoped for she stood behind me and ran her large hand down my spine like a powerful stream, all the way down to the tail, where she paused to coax out the last waves and vibrations. I felt a true liberation from surface tensions as well as deeper ones.

At other times after she had kept her hands along my shoulder blades for some time, she helped me expel the air from the lowest part of the lungs. She said that we never managed to clear that zone. I could actually feel a great relief while she was helping me and a fine inhalation every time I succeeded in freeing myself of all that old stale air that is used to nesting in those places.

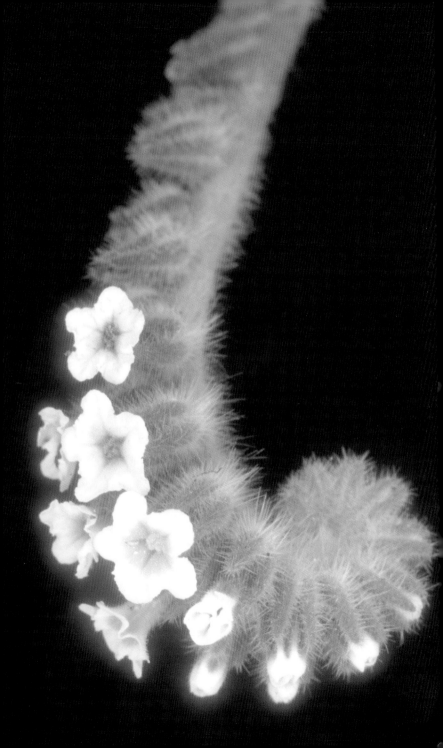

treasure house

My first years of yoga had produced a lot of confusion inside me. My attention to a constant series of directions, different ones in every single position, had created an enormous amount of uncertainty and anxiety.

In every lesson I felt projected outside myself, in order to grasp more and more instructions. In doing so, I felt dependent and weak, without the necessary tools to proceed on the yoga path by myself. On the contrary I was always in need of more detailed information.

I was very lucky then to meet Vanda, who had a great interior clarity of where to lead me. I remember how hard it was for me at the beginning to let myself go in her hands and to follow her suggestions and how I would burst into tears every time I trusted her words. I don't know how to explain how to follow this path or to choose it because Vanda took my hand firmly and lovingly from the very beginning and led me and I let myself be led. When I felt as if I had lost my way, I used to tell her of my distress. She reassured me that this was the path of the sage: to lose it in order to find it again.

We didn't talk much, because in her presence everything seemed to assume different proportions: what was insurmountable and enormous became small and what seemed minuscule and insignificant often took on a large meaning. To try to explain the relationship that links and binds a student to her teacher may be an impossible task. Every gesture seems full of feeling and understanding, every word brims with meaning, every tone of voice creates deep echoes and every phrase is heeded in order to be absorbed. Everything enhances awareness.

I remember times spent with Vanda which drew me into a place of such depth that I wished to linger there for days and days. Often, when the time for our next meeting was approaching, I would say to her: "I cannot come, I am still in the process of assimilating what happened last time." My inner space expanded in her presence to become a cave, a cavern, with resonances which continued to sound. When the intelligence enters into the heart, or perhaps the heart enters into the intelligence, wonders occur that cannot be explained because of the nature of this unique and privileged relationship.

Often I would be brimming with gratitude and say to her "What would my life have been like if I hadn't met you?" And she would respond without a moment's hesitation: "And what would I have done with mine without you?" It is a kind of love that enlarges and overflows and you have to transmit it because it leaves you so full of the wish to share with others. In the practice we get into contact with a universe that reawakens under the touch of the breath. An entire universe that repeats and refines itself in a journey from the rough and heavy towards the soft and the light. Every time we placed more attentive care to the breath, it felt like opening a door that allowed us both to enter a treasure house.

It was a vast space in semi-darkness where many precious stones were glittering. Their sparkling beauty, in time, illuminated the semi-darkness with amazing reflections of different shades.

From that treasure house I used to think that one day when she went away Vanda would take with her the jewels she so generously had given me, but when she died she was so light, she didn't seem to carry anything with her at all. She was so light that it seemed as if she was carried off by a puff of wind. Time passed and every day I was surprised to find I was still able to reconnect myself to the ground. I found that my spine, my roots and the breath were still there waiting for me to make contact. When would all this treasure vanish?

During her lifetime Vanda never asked me how I was teaching, nor what I was teaching in all those years. She often asked me if I intended to continue to teach and it almost hurt me that she felt any doubt about that. Only now, after her death, is her legacy becoming clear. The jewels. What she had shown me over such a

long period of time and what she led me to experience
have turned into splendid travelling companions,
trustworthy, honest and present in every moment of
the day. They sparkle in all their beauty when exposed
to the light of the practice. And they in turn can
be given with great generosity, and passed on with
overflowing hands.

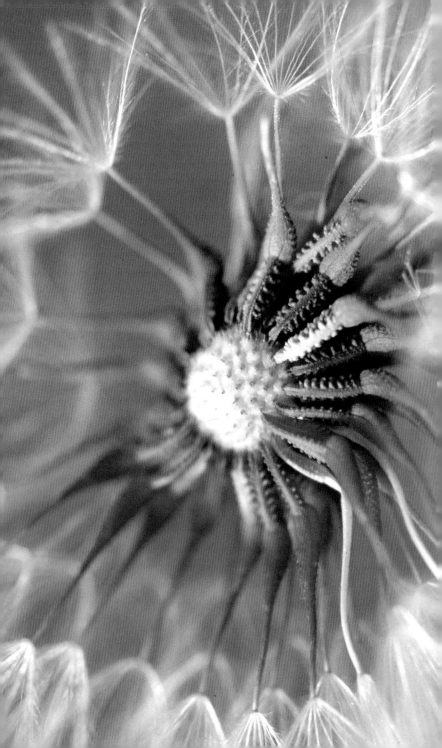

infinite time

When I first started to teach I understood only a few key points about where to focus attention. I tried to follow her exact words. I remember a week-long seminar that I gave to friends and students a few months after my first meeting with Vanda. I repeated "heels, heels, heels" over and over again, seven days in a row. They were sweet and patient with me but I suspect they experienced little else except huge feet and heavy heels.

Then it became clear to me that Vanda's words enclosed an entire universe and that she was sharing her profound experience of life. The task of all those who had studied with her and wished to transmit what they had learned was to decode her essential message so that it could be fully experienced.

It seemed vital to find words to describe the infinite series of interior events and to encourage the curiosity and keep the sense of listening active throughout the session. In a class at the beginning of the journey where everything and anything can be a distraction, this is a colossal feat – but not impossible.

Words stimulate a dialogue with the force of gravity and help to become aware of it, bringing the surrounding space more vividly into the practice. A listening state is essential to increase awareness of the presence of the breath and a series of inner awakening events.

Words link the breath, the ground, space and the spine, and bring together anything that might have lost its brilliancy. Simple language that often sounds poetic arises out of the constant discoveries that we make when we are listening and paying attention as we practise.

In a one-to-one session, the transmission is very direct. Distractions are reduced to a minimum. I was painfully aware that in a group it was crucial to find and to keep a direct contact with everyone, from the beginning to the end of the session.

Vanda spoke of eight students as an ideal number. More turned into a tribe and it made no difference then if there were twelve students or twenty-four. The risk was that the clarity would be weakened.

There is a line, like a measure for liquid that clearly marks the boundary, between being in the yoga dimension with your students or teaching them. Up to a certain number of students, guiding them feels like standing on a centre of a perennial, overflowing spring of clear water that purifies everything and everyone, as it falls. Above that number (and it is not a specific number) – as you guide the session, you have to activate something in your voice and in your presence that replaces the natural flow, and the benefits will not be the same. The magic of the small miracle that is a true yoga meeting will not be there.

From my own experience with Vanda, I felt that the

time factor, unlimited time and the possibility of following the same students for years would limit any possible weakening or distortion of her message. There was no technique to refer to, only an expansion of awareness and a reduction of effort.

If we allow ourselves to go slowly and let time spread within us, a new rhythm arises. Without any sense of urgency we approach a listening and learning attitude. Slowing down provokes an incredible resistance and releases interior tumult. But only by slowing down does time transform itself into our ally.

Awakening is what the whole being is waiting for and this is something to be aware of both as a student and as a teacher.

Touch can add a sort of instant awakening, bypassing mental activity and resistance.

Touch can arrive at places beyond the reach of words. Hands can rouse drowsy parts of the body, fingers can undo knots and tension. Touching can help to shed or get out of a heavy, coercive garment or habit. Hands moving along the spine alert us to its existence, length and its wide spectrum of movements.

Strong loving hands urge the body into a healthy and lasting contact with the ground and invite it to release and blossom into space like a flower.

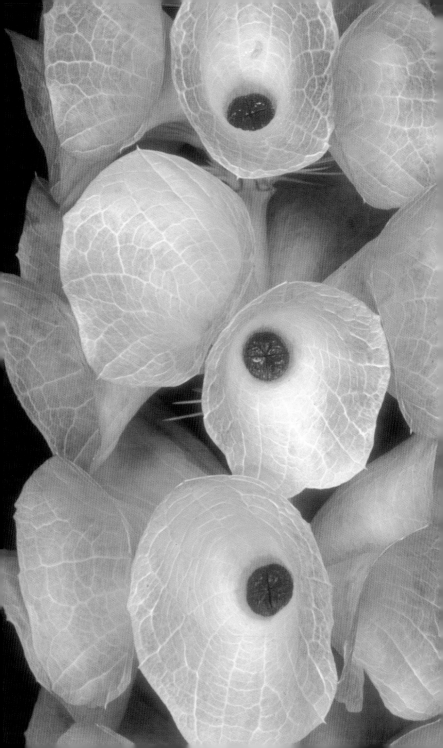

epilogue: listening

My years of studies with Vanda were spent listening together to the breath, absorbed and enthralled. Days, weeks and months where every meeting was for me the anticipation of that moment in which we would be attending to the sound of the breath, after exploring a range of positions. Silence entered the room and sitting with crossed legs in lotus position was already a precise sign that we were about to listen deeply. In that silence we would both smile, at home with the breath. The lotus position felt like a harbour which offered refuge from the open sea; it was a relief to be there.

The prevailing image was of two standing women holding a big white conch shell to their ears and listening silently to the humming sound of the sea. They are absorbed in the process of listening and do not want to let the tiniest murmuring sound escape them. Their faces are close together and a smile appears whenever they can hear that distant sound.

In the course of all the years spent with Vanda, the image has remained the same, unchanging. Then later on, the image expanded revealing the two women in their entirety.

The white garments, light layers, flutter around them, the shell always in their hands facing something invisible to all other eyes. Their lips move but no words sound. All the space around is clear and milky, their bare feet resting on white sand. The details of the shell and the expressions on their faces can still be seen. The sky grows larger, the beach longer and wider, the two women and their shell continually smaller.

Now that I have begun to write about these years, wind has blown into the image, and given movement to the clothes the women wear, and the scene sometimes fills with the indistinct colours of dawn or dusk. A breeze ruffles their clothes, and every so often they both pause to place the shell to their ears and listen.

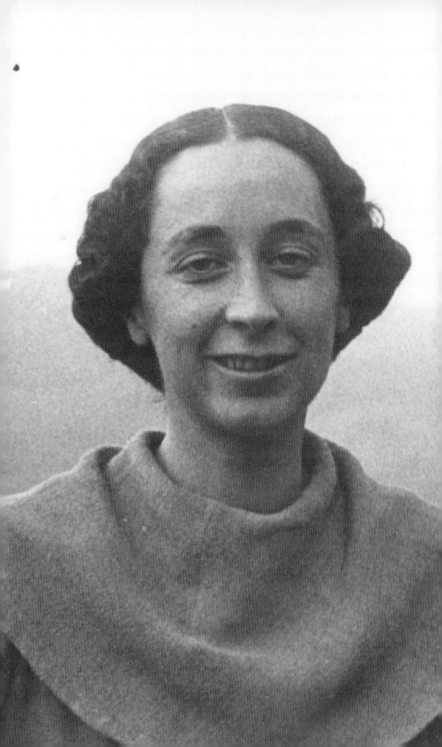

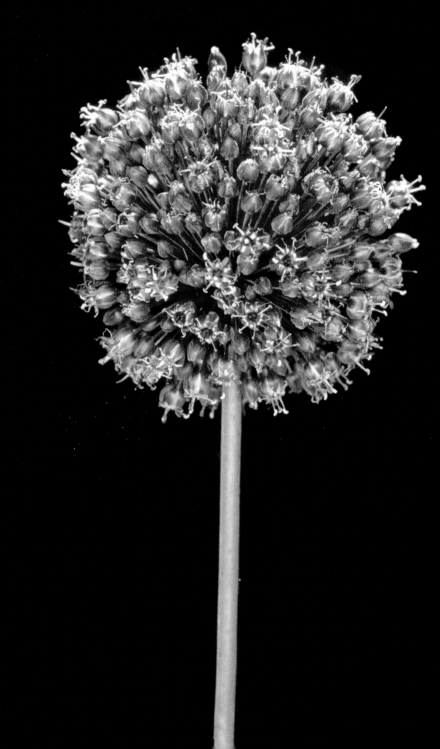

photography

All photographs, with the exception of the archive
photographs of Vanda Scaravelli on pages 6, 14 and
135, are by Dr. David Darom (ddd@mail.huji.ac.il).

cover   The Judean Desert in Bloom

p 10   Poppy, *Papaver polytrichum*

p 18   Early Morning Frost

p 24   Persian Cyclamen, *Cyclamen persicum*

p 30   Hollyhock, *Alcea dissecta*

p 34   Large Quaking Grass, *Briza maxima*

p 38   Common Caper, *Capparis spinosa*

p 44   Crown Daisy, *Chrysanthemum coronarium*

p 50   Petty Spurge, *Euphorbia peplus*

p 56   Mountain Rye, *Secale montanum*

p 60   Sea Daffodil, *Pancratium maritimum*

p 66   Globe Thistle [close up], *Echinops gaillardoti*

p 74   Ice Plant, *Mesembryanthemum crystallinum*

p 80   Bee Orchid, *Ophrys apifera*

p 84   Bulbous Meadow Grass, *Poa bulbosa*

p 88   Fragrant Heliotrope, *Heliotropium suaveolens*

p 94   Prickly Cupped Goat's Beard, *Urospermum
picroides*

p 100   Smooth Molucca Balm [dry state], *Moluccella
laevis*

p 106   Wild Leek, *Allium ampeloprasum*

acknowledgements

Thanks to Michael Eilan who almost forced me to sit down and write.

A special thank you to Michal Havkin for giving me the title of the book and putting me in touch with Dr. David Darom.

Working with David has been inspiring and fulfilling – thank you so very much.

My warmest thanks to Paola Scaravelli Cohen, Vanda's daughter, and her husband Jon Cohen for reading the manuscript over and over again and giving me invaluable suggestions.

To Ann Colcord for her precious friendship with me and Vanda that brought about this lively translation – many thanks.

I am very grateful to Jan Heron, the most empathic editor one can dream of, for her help and support.

To Martin Wagner my publisher, many many thanks for the constant trust and encouragement throughout these years.

I would like to thank all my travelling companions, yoga students and friends for keeping these memories alive.

about the author

Sandra Sabatini was born in Australia to Italian parents, grew up in Tripoli, Libya, and returned to Italy in her 20s. She started studying yoga in her early 30s, and in 1985 became a pupil of Vanda Scaravelli, author of *Awakening the Spine*.

Scaravelli died in 1999 at the age of 91. She and Sandra have introduced many teachers and students all over the world to a gentle but radical yoga that emphasizes working with the breath, gravity and the spine.

Sandra Sabatini is also the author of *Breath*, and *Autumn, Winter, Spring, Summer* (with Silvia Mori).

www.sandrasabatini.info

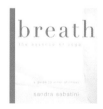

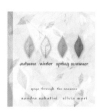

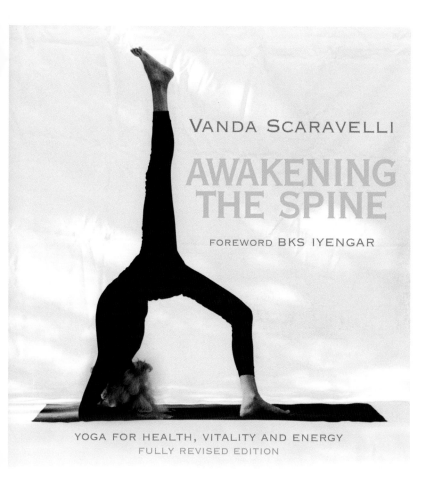